EMRO Technical Publications Series 27

Nursing and midwifery
A guide to professional regulation

World Health Organization
Regional Office for the Eastern Mediterranean
Regional Office for Europe

Cairo
2002

WHO Library Cataloguing in Publication Data

WHO Regional Office for the Eastern Mediterranean

Nursing and midwifery: a guide to professional regulation / by
WHO Regional Office for the Eastern Mediterranean and Regional
Office for Europe

    p. (WHO Technical Publications Series; 27)

    1. Nursing Administration 2. Midwifery
I. Title II. WHO Regional Office for Europe III. Series

    ISBN 92-9021-285-3   (NLM Classification: WY 105)
    ISSN 1020-0428

Cover design and layout by A. Hassanein, EMRO

Printed in Cairo, Egypt
by Alzahraa Printing for Arabic Media, 4000 copies

Contents

Foreword

Protecting the health of the public depends as much on human resources as it does on systems that are institutionalized to regulate the practice of health care providers, including nurses and midwives.

A quick review of the nursing situation in Member States in both our regions reveals that regulatory systems leave a lot to be desired. New demands for institutionalizing a comprehensive regulatory system for nursing and midwifery have been created by the health sector reform initiative and the expanding role of the private sector in health care in many countries of our regions.

This is the first joint publication between the WHO Regional Offices for the Eastern Mediterranean (EMRO) and for Europe (EURO) in the field of nursing and it represents a serious effort to strengthen nursing regulation in our regions and to develop a system to ensure the regulation of nursing practice and education. The regulatory system that would be developed would reflect the current scope of practice and would contribute to the fulfilment of the vision for nursing and midwifery entailed in the Regional Strategy for Nursing and Midwifery Development in the Eastern Mediterranean Region and in the Munich Declaration–Nurses and midwives: a force for health. Both of these regional documents call for enhancing the roles of nurses and midwives in the provision of high quality, accessible, equitable, efficient, and sensitive health services, which would ensure continuity of care and address people's rights and changing needs.

We recognize that regulation is a complex topic, but our purpose is to provide the countries with guidelines that provide direction on the process and content required for institutionalizing a comprehensive regulatory system for nursing and midwifery in Member States, based on current nursing regulation in both our regions.

We also hope that this publication will assist Member States in their efforts to develop regulatory systems, with special emphasis on increasing the capability of nurses and midwives in the area of nursing and midwifery legislation.

Guided by the World Health Assembly and Regional Committee resolutions and recommendations made by Chief Nurses, members of the Regional Advisory Panel on Nursing and Midwifery and the International Council of Nurses, this publication identifies the process and content required to institutionalize a nursing and midwifery regulatory system, to ensure the highest possible standard of nursing practice and to protect the health and safety of the public.

We hope that this publication will serve as a useful resource for policy-makers and managers in the health system, professional regulatory authorities, nurses and midwives, as well as other health professionals in their efforts to protect the health of the public and improve the quality of nursing and midwifery services.

Hussein A. Gezairy
WHO Regional Director for the Eastern
Mediterranean

Marc Danzon
WHO Regional Director for Europe

Preface

Conceive and claim a world in which regulation, as positively defined, is a powerful instrument for the good of nursing and health visiting—the world of the twenty first century. This is the vision! And this is the challenge [1].

Professional regulation of nursing and midwifery and the preparation of associated legislation is a fascinating and complex matter. Worldwide, some countries have well developed regulatory systems for nursing; others have partial or embryo systems; and still others are only just commencing discussion and debate on the issues. For those countries considering implementing a new system of professional regulation in nursing, or making changes to existing systems, the task can appear overwhelming. The wholesale importation of existing systems from other countries is rarely appropriate for a particular nation or state. It is, however, neither cost effective nor productive to ignore or duplicate work already undertaken. Valuable lessons, both positive and negative, can be learned from those who have information and experience to share. In this context, WHO commissioned this publication, as part of its commitment to empower nurses and midwives themselves to tackle issues of relevance to their own profession. It is anticipated that the information it contains will provide a useful guide to the issues which have to be considered, particularly for countries establishing regulatory systems for the first time. There is also a wealth of information here which will be useful to those countries which already have systems—whole or partial—in place.

The need for this document was originally conceived during the fourth meeting of the Regional Advisory Panel on Nursing and the consultation on nursing research priorities in the Eastern Mediterranean Region for improving quality of nursing practice and education, both held in Beirut, Lebanon, in September 1999, where professional regulation was the subject of considerable discussion and debate. The need was reaffirmed following a WHO workshop on nursing legislation held in Bratislava, Slovakia, in December 1999. It became clear that the individual countries within both the Eastern Mediterranean and European Regions of WHO[1] are moving at very different speeds in relation to regulatory processes. It also became apparent that there was not always a shared understanding of either the principles underpinning regulation or of the

---

[1]With regard to Europe, the information is targeted mainly towards those European countries which are not part of the European Union, although there will be much information here which is relevant to all.

terminology used. It was therefore agreed that a WHO guide to professional regulation in nursing and midwifery would be a useful tool to support the progress being made.

The document is not intended to be a comprehensive discourse on the conceptual basis of regulation, as that is available in other places. Rather it is designed to be a working document for those grappling with the practical realities of implementing a regulatory system in their own country or state. It offers knowledge and information, based on a range of sources and experience, on the processes of creating legislation and establishing effective regulatory systems. The target audience therefore comprises those health professionals working at the policy-making levels of ministries of health.

This guide owes a considerable debt to the work on regulation already undertaken by the International Council of Nurses and deliberately draws on Council material to avoid unnecessary duplication. There is too much to be done to waste time on doing work that has already been undertaken effectively. It is also important that as much international regulatory congruence is achieved as possible in terms of terminology, within the context of the specific needs of a particular country or region.

Acknowledgements

In accomplishing this task, many thanks are in order. Special thanks are due to members of the Eastern Mediterranean Regional Advisory Panel on Nursing and Midwifery and to the Chief Nurses in the Member States of the European Region and the Eastern Mediterranean Region who identified the need for developing regional guidelines that would provide countries with a systematic approach to developing a nursing and midwifery regulatory system. We are indebted to them for their comments and review of the manuscript. Acknowledgment is also due to Ms Maggie Wallace for her diligent work in developing the document; her input is highly appreciated by all of us.

Enaam Abou Youssef
Former Regional Adviser, Nursing and
Allied Health Personnel,
Eastern Mediterranean Region

Ainna Fawcett-Henesy
Regional Adviser for Nursing
and Midwifery
European Region

Fariba Al-Darazi
Regional Adviser, Nursing and
Allied Health Personnel,
Eastern Mediterranean Region

Guide to professional regulation

Achieving policy change

Nursing ("nursing" in this instance and throughout the document also includes midwifery) has long been influenced by a range of people. Politicians, doctors, lawyers, teachers and civil servants have all had—and in many instances still do have, to a greater or lesser extent—a significant influence on policy relating to nursing and nursing regulation, particularly nursing education. In many instances, those who have been significant by their absence in the policy debate are the nurses themselves.

Among the factors identified as impeding nursing's involvement in its own affairs are [2]: the exclusion of nurses from policy-making and decision-making at all levels in the health care system; the undervaluing of nursing, with its concomitant subordination to medicine; and sex discrimination. The latter includes the characteristics associated with work undertaken by a predominantly female workforce: low pay, low status, poor working conditions, few prospects for promotion and poor education [2]. In another study undertaken in 1999, the major obstacles to nurse involvement in decision-making, particularly at the highest level, were again identified as lack of power, inadequate education and domination of medicine. Nurses also lacked power and authority within the decision-making processes. In addition, they frequently lacked the knowledge to present proposals for decision-making [3].

Change can be difficult. It is, however, necessary if nurses are to take the initiative and seek to influence their own professional destiny. In order to influence change, three key elements are necessary: education, appropriate knowledge and accurate information upon which to base decisions. This handbook seeks to address these issues.

For significant change to occur, change in attitude is also frequently necessary on the part of those with power and influence, particularly in relation to the generosity with which information is shared within and across professions. A climate in which knowledge and information is held only by the chosen few militates against progress and the subsequent development of effective systems based on sound principles. Knowledge should be seen as a gift to be shared generously for the greater good of all those who will benefit from effective regulation. Such an approach fits in with the trend towards decentralization of health care and the associated devolution of authority and responsibility to the lowest possible levels.

The concept of regulation and the context within which it operates

The term "professional regulation" is often misunderstood and interpreted as the imposition of bureaucratic rule-bound requirements which constrain the activities of the profession concerned and serve to maintain the isolation and separateness of the professional from the person for whom they care. Nothing could be further from the truth. Professional regulation, or professional governance, as it should, perhaps, more accurately be known, should be an exciting, dynamic framework within which professional standards can be identified in order to serve the main aim of regulation—that of public protection. Good regulatory systems should be focused, flexible and enabling—ensuring that standards are comprehensive, clear, visible and achievable.

Such an approach to regulation is essential when the context within which health care is delivered is considered. The new millennium can only serve to emphasize the political, social and economic changes that are already occurring globally and that affect the delivery and organization of health care. Globalization and increase in world trade, with health care being considered as a transferable commodity; changing political and structural boundaries and the formation of new, often unusual, partnerships; increasing disparity of access to health care as the gap between the rich and the poor widens; major environmental changes bringing catastrophic damage to populations; and economic collapse affecting significant areas of the world—these are some of the issues which drive changes in the organization and delivery of health care worldwide. In addition, the effects of rapid technological change, the increasing expectations of those consuming the health services, the changing nature of employment with increased multiskilling and substitution (see glossary), an increasingly mobile international workforce, increasingly stringent resource constraints, the changing context of professional practice and the changing relationship between professionals and consumers all serve to increase the demand for innovation and flexibility on the part of the professionals. Trends towards deregulation, decentralization and devolution, together with moves towards institutional accreditation, also serve to significantly change the context within which professionals work, placing an even greater responsibility on regulatory systems to be relevant, responsive and capable of rapid evolution.

The implications of these changes for individual professionals are considerable. There is an urgent need for each individual to fully understand the changing nature of personal and professional accountability. Each individual will have to have an informed and principled understanding of their role and responsibility. They will have to be prepared to work from a basis of ethical, evidence-based practice, ready and willing to articulate the rationale for their actions and always looking for new and more effective ways of delivering good quality nursing care. Individuals will also have to be fully aware of the legal, mandatory and "custom and practice" frameworks within which their practice is set and how and when this can appropriately be adjusted, either in conjunction with other health care professionals or independently.

International initiatives

Many countries are working on new or refined systems of professional regulation, and the 1980s and 1990s saw significant activity in relation to the preparation of new regulatory legislation. In some countries (e.g. Poland and the Seychelles) this has meant the setting up of new councils/ boards or other regulatory processes. In others (e.g. France and the Philippines) specific aspects of regulation, such as codes of conduct/ethics have been devised. Nursing practice laws have also been amended in a variety of countries (e.g. Ireland, Nigeria and South Africa). Increasing emphasis has also been placed on standards for continuing professional development (e.g. United Kingdom), in recognition of the fact that qualification and/or registration is not the summit of professional endeavour but merely the start of a long professional journey in which knowledge and skills require constant renewal and updating. In some countries (e.g. Canada and the United Kingdom) where legislation relating to regulation has been in place for some time there has been a new move towards an umbrella style of regulation which incorporates all professions.

Specific initiatives within the Eastern Mediterranean and European Regions

For ease of reference, material relating specifically to the Eastern Mediterranean and European regions are included in Annexes 1 and 2 respectively.

Principles of regulation

The International Council of Nurses (ICN) set out 12 principles to be taken into consideration when developing effective professional regulation. The principles were originally set out by the Council at its meeting in 1986 [4] and were re-examined and reaffirmed in 1997 [1]. The principles related to purposefulness, relevance, definition, professional ultimacy, multiple interests and responsibilities, representational balance, professional optimacy, flexibility, efficiency and congruence, universality, fairness, and interprofessional equality and compatibility. For a detailed exposition of the principles, readers are referred to the relevant ICN documents but the author's commentary on the key points in relation to each principle is set out below. The indented text below is quoted from ICN material [1], which is reproduced with the permission of ICN.

Anyone considering the setting up of new systems of regulation, whether whole or partial, is advised to keep these principles firmly and explicitly in mind at each stage of the process and to constantly measure all activity against these benchmarks.

Principle of purposefulness: regulation should be directed towards a specific purpose

The overriding purpose of the statutory regulation of nursing is that of service to and protection of the public.

Serving and protecting the public is achieved by the delivery of competent, accessible, effective, appropriate nursing care. The regulatory body needs to be dynamic, alert and innovative in order to identify relevant changes in the policy context and the consequential changes to the organization and delivery of health care and the preparation of health care practitioners. Such a body needs to have systems in place to undertake regular critical reappraisal of practice, education and conduct/discipline systems.

Principle of relevance: regulation should be designed to achieve the stated purpose

Since the overriding purpose of statutory regulation is service to and protection of the public, the regulatory system should be designed to satisfy this intent in a comprehensive manner.

To ensure the relevance of regulatory systems there must be systems in place to ensure that there is continuous review both for organizations and individuals. There must be regular improvement in the quality and standard of care offered to patients and clients. Practice settings must constantly be monitored to ensure that they support good practice, and effective standards of education and effective assessment for both education and practice must be in place. Each aspect of regulation should be measured against this over-arching imperative; if the activity does not contribute to public protection then, although it may be valid for other purposes (e.g. improving professional status), it should not form part of a regulatory system.

Principle of definition: regulatory standards should be based upon clear definitions of professional scope and accountability

A definition of nursing and nurses should be at the heart of every system for regulation of the profession.

Nurses are responsible and accountable for nursing practice, whether they deliver care personally or by delegation to an appropriate other. There should be no room for confusion in relation to titles or roles as to which individuals are professionally qualified and which individuals are working in support of the qualified/registered staff. Where practitioners have additional specialist or advanced competencies this should also be made clear to those for whom they care. Whilst there should be a clear definition of the role and boundaries of practice, it should be recognized that all professional practice evolves over time according to the state of knowledge and other social, political or economic circumstances. Interprofessional boundaries are also increasingly fluid depending on the knowledge base and skill mix of the various professionals available.

In addition, it is imperative that all individuals working in a professional capacity recognize and honour their personal, professional accountability. As such, they must ensure that they have the knowledge and skills required to deliver effective care at all times. Continuing professional development mechanisms must be in place in order for individuals to demonstrate that they are maintaining and developing their professional knowledge and competence throughout their careers.

Principle of professional ultimacy: regulatory definition and standards should promote the fullest development of the professional commensurate with its potential social contribution

Since the function of a profession is, by definition, to serve society, nursing, in common with other health professions, should be encouraged to serve to its maximum capability.

This principle is particularly important in cultures where, for whatever reason, nursing has adopted or been relegated to a subordinate position. Individual nurses and the profession as a whole must seek to be the agents of constructive change, not merely the passive recipients of change determined by others. The nursing voice, based on effective research evidence, must be heard as a key influencer on all health policy issues. Nursing education must be designed to help to harness an articulate and well considered approach to the policy context within which nursing is delivered and nurses must expect to be influential and take their equal place at the policy table along with other health care professionals on the basis of the significant contribution that they can make.

Principle of multiple interest and responsibilities: regulatory systems should recognize and incorporate the legitimate roles and responsibilities of interested parties, the public, the profession and its members, government, employers and other professions in various aspects of standard setting and administration

It is the responsibility of the profession to take the leading role in its professional governance.

Professional self-regulation must be the responsibility of the profession concerned, both of its individual members and collectively. However, such a lead role must be tempered by genuine and explicit recognition of the legitimate role played by others. The involvement of other parties, particularly and increasingly those who are the recipients of care, is vital for public protection policies to be seen as relevant and responsive. It is for the profession to provide, through a genuine and comprehensive consultation process, the standards by which it will be measured and against which its members will be held accountable. Such standards should include those for education, conduct, service requirements, knowledge and skills and practice advances. It is not for nursing to passively receive these standards as a result of decisions made on its behalf by others.

Principle of representational balance: the design of the regulatory system should acknowledge and appropriately balance interdependent interests

It is not in the best interests of any profession to be unchallenged in its regulatory standard and processes.

To complement the previous principle, this makes it clear that no profession should be entirely free in managing its own regulation, for in that there lies a real danger of indulgent self-interest, lack of accountability and subsequent and catastrophic loss of public confidence. All those parties with legitimate interests should have explicit and visible roles and no one profession should be seen to dominate others. Neither should government influence inappropriately dominate the professions. Professional boundaries and actual and potential conflict of interests will need to be the subject of regular and considered debate among the relevant bodies. Where professions do not properly honour this principle, then sooner or later there will be a significant challenge to the power of that profession, with resultant loss of confidence and consequential damage to the concept of professional regulation.

Principle of professional optimacy: regulatory systems should provide and be limited to those controls and restrictions necessary to achieve their objectives

The purpose of statutory regulation is to ensure that competent and accessible care is available from accountable professionals and this should be done using efficient, effective and economic processes.

There is a real danger in establishing new regulatory systems, (especially where legislation has been slow in coming and hard won) of seeking to place too much emphasis on the details of regulatory systems and not paying enough attention to the underpinning principles. Such an approach is short-sighted and will, sooner or later, prove to be self-defeating in that standards will be difficult and slow to change and will rapidly lack relevance and responsiveness. Focus should be on the important issues such as mandatory credentialling and continuing professional development, the accreditation of those with additional qualifications, the effective management of those who support nurses, the positive management of poor practice and effective disciplinary processes. Careful consideration should be given to the way in which goals are achieved; not all standards, for example, need to be set in legislation—some may be equally effective if they are advisory.

Principle of flexibility: standards and processes of regulation should be sufficiently broad and flexible to achieve their objective and at the same time permit freedom for innovation, growth and change

Regulation should be neither too general nor too specific. Scope of practice definitions and educational standards should give broad guidance to practitioners and employers through general statements of nursing function.

As highlighted in some of the previous discussions it is important that standards are expressed as flexibly as is compatible with clarity and effectiveness. This will enable response to innovation, changes in practice and the delivery of care and the changing expectations of those to whom care is given. Broad guidance should be the goal, rather than detailed prescription. Such an approach should ensure that nurses are capable of responding to changes in their practice environment while still working safely and effectively from an evidence base. This is particularly important as nursing skills become more transferable, nurses become evermore mobile and international movement increases every year. Consideration should be given to the form in which guidance is best given to achieve the objective of good care; working from sound principles is much safer that working from a rigid set of rules.

Principle of efficiency and congruence: regulatory systems should operate in the most efficient manner ensuring coherence and coordination among their parts

Regulatory activity on behalf of all interested parties should be coordinated to accomplish the purpose of regulation in a streamlined and uniform manner.

Given that by their nature regulatory systems involve a number of different bodies, both within a country or state and frequently beyond, it is important that there is maximum coordination of all the relevant parts. While ideally, systems should be established as a congruent whole, the reality is that most systems evolve over time on a piecemeal basis. This can lead to fragmentation and may result either in duplication of activity or in vital elements of a process being omitted. This is particularly the case where different responsibilities are vested in different bodies, especially if relationships between the parties are not good and power and/or control is sought by one at the expense of another. It can also be a problem within the same organization if effective systems are not in place to ensure congruence and comparability

Principle of universality: regulatory systems should promote universal standards of performance and foster professional identity and mobility to the fullest extent compatible with local need and circumstances

Although some recognition must be given to local need and cultural differences, substantial inconsistency is antithetical to the achievement of broad and uniform development of the profession and free movement of practitioners.

As discussed within the principle of flexibility, it is ideal if regulatory systems are as universal as possible. Nursing (and indeed health care generally) is an increasingly mobile commodity, with the real possibility of both patients and nurses moving across national boundaries. If patients travel for care, for example a specific operation, it is important that the nursing care is of a standard to support the patients' nursing needs in every way. Whilst recognizing and honouring country-specific needs and approaches, such application should be from as universal a base as possible, so that nurses and nursing have a common set of baseline competencies, incorporating both knowledge, skills and attitudes, for effective practice, wherever they may be delivered.

Principle of fairness: processes should provide honest and just treatment for those parties regulated

Honest and just systems of regulation must be visible, open and objective with explicit routes for appeal.

This principle is very clear, yet it is not one which has been adhered to in a number of existing systems. All the standards and processes of any regulatory system must be explicitly visible, so that individuals know what they are trying to achieve and, where they are not successful, for what reason they have not met the required standard. Standards need to be well publicized and explicit. They also need to be specifically scrutinized to ensure that they are not overtly or covertly discriminatory on any grounds.

Principle of interprofessional equality and compatibility: in standards and processes, regulatory systems should recognise the equality and interdependence of professions offering essential services.

For professions to develop and work collaboratively on the public behalf, education and practice standards need to be comparable and regulatory processes complementary.

Nursing is an integral part of health care, and should have standards and processes which are comparable to those of other health care colleagues. This applies to all elements of any regulatory system, including standards for education, practice and conduct. This does nor necessarily mean, for instance, that education programmes have to be of the same length but they should be of a similar quality, expecting the highest standards of their students in a comparable education setting. Standards for discipline or conduct should be comparable for all health care professions; different treatment of different professionals who have been involved in the same or similar incidents is not acceptable, either in terms of justice or of public protection.

Establishing a regulatory system

Establishing a comprehensive regulatory system requires the completion of a number of steps. Ideally any new system should be considered as an integrated whole. In reality however few countries start from nothing; usually some work will already have been done and will need to be incorporated in some way into a new system. Whether starting a new system or modifying an existing one, it will be helpful to consider the following steps, if only to ensure that nothing has been left out. In practice, various elements of the process will need adjusting to accommodate the needs of country concerned and will assume greater or lesser importance depending upon the particular circumstances.

1. Determining a policy

First of all a clear policy needs to be agreed by the body/bodies with responsibility for such. This may be the nursing association, government, the nursing council/board or other body. Policy should be established through a process of formal and informal consultation if it is to be effectively put into practice. If the key players (who need to be carefully and comprehensively identified) are not involved in the process then the policy is likely to be unsuccessful. Consultation will not, of course, mean that everyone can have their own way; compromises will still have to be made but frank discussion of the options and the reasons for the final decisions will help those decisions to be better understood and accepted.

Ideally the total policy should relate to a comprehensive regulatory system even if implementation will take place on an incremental basis, depending on issues such as resources and infrastructure changes. In this way different elements can be worked on at different rates; for example, work could be done on preparing a code of conduct while also considering changes to licence-to-practise requirements. If an existing system is used for a model, care should be taken to ensure that the final scheme is professionally, socially, economically and culturally appropriate to the setting in which it is to be used.

2. Determining a strategy

Once the policy is agreed, a clear and explicit strategy and plan of action should be confirmed which encompasses all the elements of the policy from its inception to its final implementation. For ultimate success, it is vital that the implementation phase be given as much time and as many resources as the policy phase. The responsibility for implementing the total strategy and the separate phases/elements of the action plan should be clear, and lines of accountability should be explicit and visible. Good communication is essential to success, and time and effort should be given to ensuring that proposed changes are understood by all those who will be affected.

3. Identifying the key players

For policy change to be successful it is necessary to win as many hearts and minds as possible in advance of implementation. It is vital to consider everyone who may have a legitimate role. This may include, for example:

*   nursing associations/organizations
*   influential groups, e.g. managers, educationalists
*   government
*   the public
*   patients' representatives
*   other professions
*   voluntary groups
*   other relevant/influential bodies

Attention should also be given to identifying and cultivating influential individuals who may be helpful in terms of achieving significant policy change, especially where there may be some opposition.

4. Consultation (formal and informal)

Effective consultation processes are essential if the eventual policy is to have the goodwill and support of those affected. The ultimate operational success of the policy may well depend on the effectiveness of the consultation process. While it is clearly unlikely that all interested parties will be equally pleased with the policy outcomes, at least if an opportunity has been given for them to have their say and an explanation offered as to why certain decisions were made, goodwill will have been maintained.

If a policy-making body already exists, the requirements for formal consultation may already be well established. In some instances the process may be set down within existing legislation and the organizations which have to be consulted will be explicitly defined. Alternatively, there may be a general phrase to the effect that consultation must take place with all those organizations or individuals who may be affected, actually or potentially, by any changes. Any formal consultation process should be regularly reviewed as "interested parties" are likely to change significantly over time. The increased involvement of consumers and/or patient representatives is a good example of a significant change in the past decade.

In addition to honouring any formal consultation process, the informal processes are equally important, although they may not be as visible. Influential opinion formers, such as politicians, key health care managers and professionals, should be identified and lobbied by all appropriate means. Such activity is essential in terms of achieving significant policy change.

Preparation of legislation

The prerequisite for good primary legislation is a clear and workable policy. This is not always as obvious as it sounds. Where the policy position is likely to be contentious, it is important to gain as much support from those who will be affected by the legislation as possible before the process of law gets under way. In this way the possibility of any challenge to the legislation and the consequential slowing down or, worse, the aborting of the process, can be avoided, or at least minimized. A good consultation process during the policy-making stage is therefore essential. (See "Establishing a regulatory system", item 4 above.)

Once the policy has been agreed the preparation of the legislation to put that policy into effect can begin. Preparing effective legislation requires good cooperation between the policy-makers and those responsible for drafting the legislation. It is not always easy, indeed it is not always possible, to translate policy intent into legislation. Compromises frequently have to be made but they should be carefully negotiated to ensure that the final act or rules are acceptable in both policy and operational terms. The process should be managed by representatives of those who fully understand the policy intent and its intended operation, together with those who will actually draft the legislation. Each element of the legislation should be subject to scrutiny to ensure that its operation is feasible, realistic and cost–effective.

It should not be forgotten that legislation affecting other professions, such as the prescribing of medicines, frequently has an effect on nursing activity and this fact should not be overlooked when new nursing legislation is planned.

Primary legislation (the act) will be the main benchmark from which all else flows. The act will be the framework for the specific piece of legislation. Primary legislation is normally slow, cumbersome and expensive to change and should therefore be drafted to ensure that it is capable of interpretation which may evolve in response to changing circumstances. For example, in relation to regulation, the act may give the regulatory body the power to "provide advice". It would be unhelpful and unnecessarily restrictive to describe the nature of that advice which, in any case, is likely to change over time and in response to differing circumstances.

Secondary legislation (known as rules, statutory instruments or orders) must always have its origins in the primary legislation. It is possible to change secondary legislation more easily and quickly than primary legislation, although it will still be a rigorous and time-consuming process

Development of a nursing practice act

A comprehensive regulatory system will need a firm basis. Much of this basis will need to be legislative. Legislation will provide structure, support and a clear imperative in relation to policy. Standards set in legislation have to be fulfilled. The structure of a new system must therefore be underpinned by primary legislation—a nursing practice act—as this is the source for the regulatory body's standard-setting powers. Secondary legislation (statutory instruments or rules), will be used for putting the detail on to the standards. For example, the act will give the body the power to make rules in relation to education criteria. The rules will then give further detail in respect of the type of criteria required.

While legislation is extremely powerful, it should also be remembered that producing or changing legislation, particularly primary legislation, is usually a slow, cumbersome and expensive process, not to be embarked upon lightly. Serious consideration should therefore always be given to whether the policy objective could be as effectively met by other means. For example, this could be, by means of a mandate from a significant body, such as a professional organization or statutory regulatory body. Alternatively, some standards, such as a code of conduct, may be as effective providing that the code's power to give advice is in the primary legislation. Such an approach has the advantage of comparative ease of alteration, to reflect changes in practice and the organization of care.

The following may serve as a guide.

Primary legislation

As a minimum, one would expect to see the following within a nursing practice act:

* description of the purpose and scope of the regulatory body
* establishment and composition of the regulatory body
* method of appointment/election to the regulatory body
* structure and organization of the regulatory body
* a definition of nursing, the nursing role and the categories/level of nurse
* standards for pre-qualifying/registration education
* standards for achieving registration/licensure
* standards for maintaining registration/licensure
* standards for practice
* the position of those not covered by the act, e.g. nursing assistants
* the authority given to the regulatory body to set standards (e.g. for education, registration, licensure, practice)
* the authority given to the regulatory body to issue rules and regulations
* the authority given to the regulatory body to collect fees

Secondary legislation

Secondary legislation may address standards such as the following:

Education standards
* entry criteria, e.g. age, academic level/qualifications, length/level of schooling
* length/balance of theory and practice
* breaks in practice
* academic level of qualification
* competencies for different levels of nurse
* final qualification

Registration/licence to practise standards
* criteria for registration/licence to practise
* criteria for maintaining registration/licence to practise
* criteria for losing registration/licence to practise

Practice standards

- code of conduct/ethics as a baseline for practice
- scope of practice defined
- practice standards

Education following qualification standards

- specialist/advanced qualifications/certification, e.g. clinical management, teaching
- specific additional qualifications for practice in certain areas
- continuing professional development requirements for maintaining registration
- designation and definition of specialist and auxiliary personnel standards

Discipline/conduct standards

- What will be the benchmark against which misconduct will be judged? For example, a code of conduct/ethics or a broad definition of misconduct
- What will be the mechanism for investigation? It will need to be visible and fair, with specific appeal mechanisms
- What sanctions will be available for misconduct? For example, caution, suspension, removal from register/right to practise
- What reinstatement process is there to be?

Policy change checklist

When considering policy change, the following check list will be helpful.

- Do you have a clear policy to implement?
- Do you have a strategy/action plan?
- Have you identified all the key players?
- Have you consulted all the key players during the process?
- Do you have an implementation strategy?
- Do you have an information strategy?
- Check again. Have you consulted everyone necessary, both formal and informal?
- Are there any particular individuals who need targetting?
- Do you need new/amended legislation to implement any new policies?
- Are you sure that the legislation can deliver your policy objectives?
- Is the infrastructure in place to support any new systems?
- Is a communication strategy in place which will reach all those affected by any changes?
- Do you need a help-line to explain any new policies?

Time-frame

The time-frame for the design and implementation of any regulatory system will depend upon the particular circumstance of the country/state concerned. It will be affected, for example, by whether a complete system is being designed from the beginning or whether elements are already in place. However, that said, the following time-line may be helpful as a guide:

6–12 months	3–6 months	3 months	12 months	variable
work starts on formulating a policy	consultation on proposals	refining of policy	preparation of legislation	implementation of policy
		preparation of infrastructure		

Glossary

The glossary is based substantially on that used by the International Council of Nurses and is reproduced with the permission of ICN. Items marked with an * have been added by the author at the request of delegates to the meetings referred to in the preface.

Advanced nursing practice

Practice by nurses who, having acquired the knowledge base and clinical competencies for specialization, also possess the depth and breadth of knowledge and competencies to an extent warranting an expanded and more autonomous scope of practice. In most cases a graduate education is a requirement.

Competence

A level of performance demonstrating the effective application of knowledge, skill and judgement.

Continuing education or continuing professional development (CPD)

The whole range of learning activities, from the time of initial qualification until retirement, undertaken by the individual for the benefit of improving the health of the public and professional development.

Continuing education credit (unit, contact hour or point)

A unit of measure that gives a value to an approved organized continuing education learning activity, theoretical or practical.

Credentialling

A term applied to processes used to designate that an individual, programme, institution or product have met established standards set by an agent (governmental or nongovernmental) recognized as qualified to carry out this task. The standard may be minimal and mandatory or above the minimum and voluntary. Licensure, registration, accreditation, approval, certification, recognition or endorsement may be used to describe different credentialling processes but this terminology is not used consistently across different settings and countries. Credentials are marks or "stamps" of quality and achievement communicating to employers, payers and consumers what to expect from a credentialled nurse, specialist, course, programme of study, institution of higher education, hospital or health service, or health care products, technology, or device. Credentials may be periodically renewed as a means of assuring continued standards of competence and they may be withdrawn when standards of competence or behaviour are no longer met.

Governance

Governance, meaning the process of controlling or guiding the profession, is preferred by some who find the word **regulation** restrictive and legalistic. See **Regulation**.

Health for all

A level of health that will permit individuals, families and communities to lead socially and economically productive life.

Institutional licensing

The institution, having complied with government regulation, determines the scope of practice for each worker, and does not need to consider limitations mandated by practice acts defining roles, qualifications, and job standards for individual health professions. Instead each licensed institution would be the agent to define roles, qualifications and standards for the individual health professions.

Legislation*

Law(s) or the process of making law. Primary legislation refers to government acts and defines broad powers. Secondary legislation (rules, orders) defines further details of the powers enshrined in primary legislation.

Licensure*

The granting through statute, by a government body, of authority to practise a profession and to use an exclusive title, to persons who meet established standards of education and competence. Sometimes used synonymously (and often inaccurately) with the term **registration** (see **Registration**).

Mandatory regulation	A term usually applied when the authority for regulation is governmental and approval for practice is required. Standards are usually set at the minimum required for public protection.
Multiskilling	A combination of skills derived from several work areas.
Nursing practice act*	The legislation which underpins the structure, processes and outcomes of nursing (and/or midwifery) regulation, usually incorporating the structure and functions of the regulatory body/ies and standards for education, practice and discipline/conduct.
Nurse specialist	A nurse prepared beyond the level of a nurse generalist and authorized to practise as a specialist with advanced expertise in a branch of the nursing field. Speciality practice includes clinical teaching, administration, research and consultant roles. Post-basic nursing education for speciality practice is a formally recognized programme of study built on the general education of the nurse and providing the content and the experience to ensure competency in speciality practice.
Omnibus or **umbrella legislation**	A broad single act that encompasses a number of individual practice acts. The broader statutes form the umbrella legislation under which each licensing authority must work. Different models of omnibus legislation exist.
Policy*	A course or principle of action adopted or proposed by a significant body, organization, government, etc.
Professional regulation*	An umbrella term which should incorporate reference to all the structures, processes and outcomes associated with the governance of a profession. Often and inaccurately used in a narrow, reductionist sense, solely in relation to professional discipline.

Registration*   Entry of a name on a professional register, after meeting
                           certain standards of education and/or practice. Usually a
                           requirement for professional practice. Not necessarily
                           synonymous with **licensure** (see **Licensure**).

Regulation   All of those legitimate and appropriate means
                           (governmental, professional, private and individual)
                           whereby order, identity, consistency and control are
                           brought to the profession. The profession and its members
                           are defined; the scope of practice is determined; standards
                           of education and of ethical and competent practice are set;
                           and systems of accountability are established through these
                           means (see **Governance**).

Regulatory system*   All the mechanical structures associated with the
                           regulation of a profession. A variety of different systems
                           can achieve effective regulation, albeit based on similar
                           principles.

**Reserved or restricted   Tasks or services that are reserved exclusively to one
acts**   health profession (or shared jointly with another). This is
                           usually done because of risks of harm to the health and
                           well-being associated with the task or service.

Scope of practice   The range of activities that can be carried out by a nurse. It
                           defines the limits of practice of a licensed/registered nurse.

Self-governance   The governance of nurses and nursing by nurses in the
                           public interest.

Self-regulation   See **Self-governance**.

Standard   The desirable and achievable level of performance against
                           which actual practice is compared.

Statutory regulation   A term applied to regulation that is mandated by a law, act,
                           decree or statute.

Strategy*   A plan of action or policy.

Substitution   Replacing the expensive commodity, service or person with an equally effective cheaper equivalent or replacing the less effective with the more effective.

Support workers (nursing)   This term refers to all unlicensed assistive personnel engaged in nursing activities.

Telemedicine   The provision of health care using interactive audio, visual and data communication. It includes the delivery of care, consultations, diagnosis, counselling, advice and treatment, as well as the transfer of data. To a certain extent, telemedicine is a substitute for face-to-face contact between the health care provider and the client and between health care providers themselves. The terms **telenursing** and **telehealth** may also be used.

Voluntary regulation   This refers to regulation that is conducted by an authority external to the government. The credential or qualification thus earned is not required for practice or the service to be rendered.

References

1. *ICN on regulation: towards 21st century models.* Geneva, International Council of Nurses, 1997.

2. Salvage J, Heijnen S, eds. *Nursing in Europe: a resource for better health.* Copenhagen, WHO Regional Office for Europe (WHO Regional Publications, European Series, No. 74), 1997.

3. *Nursing and midwifery in the 21st century. Survey on nursing practice, management, education and research in Europe.* Helsinki, Finland, Ministry of Social Affairs and Health, 1999.

4. *Report on the regulation of nursing.* Geneva, International Council of Nurses, 1986.

5. Affara FA, Styles MM. *A nursing regulation guidebook: from principle to power.* Geneva, International Council of Nurses, 1992.

Further reading

Pyne RH, ed. *Professional discipline in nursing, midwifery and health visiting*, 3rd ed. Oxford, Blackwell Science, 1997.

WHO Regional Committee for the Eastern Mediterranean. *The need for national planning for nursing and midwifery in the Eastern Mediterranean Region.* 1994 (resolution EM/RC41/R.10).

WHO Regional Committee for the Eastern Mediterranean. *Improving the quality of nursing and midwifery in the Eastern Mediterranean Region.* 1998 (resolution EM/RC45/R.12).

Wallace MJ. *Lifelong learning: PREP in action.* Edinburgh, Churchill Livingstone, 1999.

Regulatory mechanisms for nurse training and practice: meeting primary health care needs. Report of a WHO Study Group. Geneva, World Health Organization, 1986 (World Health Organization Technical Report Series, No. 738).

World Health Assembly. *Strengthening nursing and midwifery.* 1996 (resolution WHA49.1).

World Health Assembly. *The role of health research.* 1990 (resolution WHA43.19).

Annex 1

Current situation in the Eastern Mediterranean Region

There is a wide range of activity and of progress within the Eastern Mediterranean Region in relation to varying aspects of professional regulation. Five countries (Bahrain, Cyprus, Lebanon, Pakistan and Sudan) have nursing practice acts. Valid updated registration systems are available in Bahrain and in the United Arab Emirates, and Saudi Arabia has a registration system in place for overseas nationals only. No countries have yet implemented a code of conduct/ethics, although relevant work is underway in some areas, such as Cyprus, Jordan, Sudan and Palestine. Aspects of work on quality systems, such as scope of practice, national standards for nursing practice and protocols of care have been undertaken by some countries, such as Bahrain, Morocco, Jordan, Qatar and United Arab Emirates. A number of countries (Bahrain, Cyprus, Djibouti, Jordan, Oman, Qatar, Saudi Arabia, Syrian Arab Republic, United Arab Emirates and Republic of Yemen) have adopted international and WHO recommendations to upgrade entrance requirements for basic nursing education to completion of secondary education. More specific examples are set out below. It is stressed however that these are not intended to represent a comprehensive picture of all regulatory activity in the Region.

Jordan

There are two laws that pertain to nursing and midwifery practice. The first is the Health Professional Licensing Law, which requires health professionals to register in the Ministry of Health before practising their profession. Follow-up of those who do not register is inadequate however. The law does not require continuing education for relicensing. The second law, which relates to the Jordanian Nurses and Midwives Council, was passed by Parliament in July 1999. All nurses and midwives in Jordan should register with the Council. It is considered by experts within the country that both laws are in need of review and revision to reflect the changing health care and nursing needs of the population.

Bahrain

In the past decade Bahrain has enacted a statute that regulates the registration and licensure of nurses and midwives. Although the statute is enacted as part of an umbrella law covering the allied health professions, nursing and midwifery, each profession had its own implementing resolution. A computerized system of nursing and midwifery registration has also been developed, with the technical support of WHO. In addition, a system for assessment of applications for nursing and midwifery has been put into place. Employers are involved in the process of relicensure of nurses.

United Arab Emirates

Between 1996 and 1998 the Department of Nursing, with technical support from WHO, and working through a committee, was given a remit to organize the practice of the nursing profession and draft a nursing act. The committee had representatives from a range of disciplines, including the military services, the private sector, and nursing schools and colleges. A comprehensive consultation process took place to ensure that the draft legislation is congruent with other national legislation.

Cyprus

On an initiative from within the profession, and working together with the government, nursing legislation was enacted in 1988. The enactment of the law ensures that clients and communities are cared for by appropriately educated and qualified nurses and midwives. The legislation is similar to that for other health care professionals, e.g. physicians and pharmacists. Admission to the professional register (based on meeting specific standards for education and conduct and references) which gives the right to practice, is the responsibility of the Nursing and Midwifery Council. In addition, in order to practise as a nurse or midwife in Cyprus an individual is required to be a member of the Cyprus Nurses Association. The Association selects four nurses every two years to serve on the Nursing and Midwifery Council, together with five appointed by the Ministry of Health and one registrar. Of the five, one must practise in general nursing, one in psychiatric nursing, one in nursing education, one must be a health visitor and one a practising midwife.

Annex 2

Current situation in the European Region

Gathering accurate information about existing systems of professional regulation throughout Europe is not easy. Common systems are not in place and resources are limited. Differing terminology, differing ways of collecting information (where it is collected at all), differing cultural perspectives, changing situations and disparate professional structures, in addition to the difficulties imposed by the process of translation, all impede the process of accurate data collection. The information presented here is intended to be illustrative of activity and makes no attempt to be an exhaustive description of the current state of regulation systems in Europe. For a more detailed description readers are directed towards the nursing and midwifery profiles of each country, which are available on the website of the Regional Office for Europe www.euro.who.int.

All European countries have legislation of some kind to determine the practice of the health care professions. The nature and breadth of the legislation and its relevance to professional education and practice and the current delivery of health care varies widely. Given that any division is arbitrary, the following information has been broadly divided into the situation within the central and eastern European countries (CEE)/newly independent states (NIS) and the European Union (EU)/European Free Trade Area (EFTA), for practical purposes described here as CEE/NIS and EU/EFTA. This is because in the countries of the EU a significant part of the professional regulation for nursing and midwifery, that of education, is determined by European Union directives. This provides a common benchmark, which to a degree offers a minimum standard, which is frequently not present outside the EU. It is also a standard to which many non-EU countries aspire. The Council of Europe (CE) has also made a number of recommendations[2] relating to aspects of professional regulation, such those relating to continuing education.

---

[2]European Health Committee Working Party on the Role and Education of Nurses. *The role and education of nurses*, Strasbourg, Council of Europe, 1994.

CEE/NIS Europe

Even if accurate up-to-date information is difficult to collect, it is clear that many countries are seeking to move forward on various aspects of professional regulation. For example, in the last decade changes have been or are being made to nursing education in the Czech Republic, Latvia, Slovenia and Romania. Yugoslavia (Serbia and Montenegro) is currently looking at changes to professional education to move towards a higher education system. Slovakia is considering the preparation of a nursing practice act. Work on the codification of ethical principles for nurses and the role of the nurse is under way in Lithuania. A revision of the existing health law in Hungary in 1997 now defines, for the first time, nursing, the scope of nursing and nursing practice. In addition, most NIS countries are updating their legislation, to replace the old Public Health Law of the former USSR. Registration and licensure requirements throughout the area vary considerably, with most countries having no integrated comprehensive system but an increasing number of countries considering the implementation of some sort of system or with embryo systems being developed. Some countries, such as Hungary, also have formal requirements for the renewal of licensure on a five-yearly basis.

EU/EFTA Europe

Within the EU, the scope and content of regulation-related legislation varies considerably, from detailed legislative practice requirements, such as that for nursing in Norway, to guidance by broad principles set out in codes of conduct or ethics. The majority of western European countries have some form of registration system with varying forms of licensure. Greece, for example, requires by law that an individual must possess a degree from a state-recognized institution, together with a licence from the local municipality department of hygiene, in order to practise as a nurse. In addition to initial licensure, statutory updating requirements are also in place in some countries, such as the United Kingdom. Finland requires individuals to register in the Central Register of Health Service Professionals to acquire the right to practise, and the right to use a professional title is also linked to registration.

However, within the EU the standards for professional nursing and midwifery education are quite explicit, having been harmonized across the member countries, and are laid down in the EU directives for nurses responsible for general care (77/452/EEC and 77/453/EEC)[3] and those for midwives (80/154/EEC and 80/155/EEC).[4] Countries seeking to join the EU will be required by law to meet the standards set out in these directives. The directives are "managed" by advisory committees for the professions

---

[3]*Official journal of the European Communities*, 1977, 20:L176.

[4]*Official journal of the European Communities*, 1980, 23:L33.

concerned. For example, the Advisory Committee on Training in Nursing is currently undertaking work on specialist practice and describing competency-based outcomes for general nursing.

A key objective of the directives is to facilitate freedom of movement for those individuals who are nationals of member states and who have completed recognized certification. Individuals who have undertaken a programme of education which meets the directives' requirements, are entitled to be registered, or licensed to practise, in another member state on application to that country's competent authority (the body with the power to register practitioners). While registration does not guarantee a work permit or employment, it is the first essential part of the process of seeking to practise one's profession in another country.